Deep Fat Loss

by Ginger Gerred

- Fat has been the cause of many health problems
- Fat often causes inflammation and many other diseases.
- Inflammation is a precursor to cancer
- Inflammation is just one of the many symptoms of joint pain
- Excessive weight can cause degenerative disease
- Degenerative Disease can also be categorized as a form or type of arthritis

We hope to help you find natural and easy remedies to reduce or eliminate fat from your deep tissue around your organs and begin a healthier and longer life.

This book is a personal home health care guide

that has the best information on how to eliminate

deep fat loss. We hope for you to journal

personal notes on or on each page for you to

write in your own preferences, recipes or other

tips that help you or your family members.

Use it like a living health journal of recipes and

remedies for your family's home health care.

 In this edition of "Deep Fat Loss" we recommend

that you drink lots of water, keep a daily food

journal and eat lots of green leafy vegetables.

Drink lots of teas (especially green) and use lots of spices in your foods. And if you like ginger and cinnamon then you may even try both in your tea. It is a good idea to stay away from red meats, prepackaged foods, sugars, sweets (unless sweetened with a healthy substitute) and eat an apple a day too.

Weight loss & Fat reduction:

One of the latest discoveries on "Deep Fat Loss" is

a Jiaogulan Tea or Gynostemma pentaphyllum. It

not only promotes longevity with its adaptogens

& antiaging properties but most of all it is one of

the leading "Deep Fat" reducers available. Find it

here: www.tinyurl.com/DeepFatLoss

Chromium Picolinate fights certain types of

diabetes. Acai Berry

Tonalin CLA (Safflower Oil is where some CLA comes from) reduces belly fat in women rich in anti-oxidants

Green Tea helps curb appetite, burn calories and full of cancer fighting nutrients.

African Mango reduces belly fat. And Drugs.com says "Research on African mango shows beneficial effects for diabetes and obesity, as well as analgesic, antimicrobial, antioxidant" www.Drugs.com

Alpha Lipoic Acid fights against neuropathy

Vinegar helps cleans the body of yeast

Kelp helps fight against virus' when combined

with B Complex

Ginseng for added energy and stress relief

Aloe Vera Gel great for constipation and for

enzymatic therapy.

Konjac fiber that makes you feel full Push away

from the table a little take a walk or swim 30

minutes a day.

Hoodia Gardenia greatly suppresses the appetite.

Green Tea Weight Loss Program (Click Image To

Order)

Type 2 Diabetes control:

Garcinia Cambogia

Hoodia Gardenia

Gynostemma or Jiaogulan

African Mango

Chromium picolinate

Pine Nut

Tonalin CLA

Acai Berry

Green Tea

Alpha Lipoic Acid

Apple Cider Vinegar

Kelp B Complex

Ginseng

Aloe Vera Gel

Konjac (fiber that makes you feel full) Push away

from the table a little take ride on a bike, a walk or

swim 30 minutes a day.

This is a compilation of over 16 years of my

personal self-study and University level studies.

As new information from new research presents

new data and new statistics we will continue to

update our readers on the latest treatments and

discoveries.

All Vitamin and Supplement doses are to be taken

as the label on the brand of your choice of

purchase recommends unless otherwise stated by

your doctor. Dosages for specific illnesses of

cancer or arthritis are to be taken as suggested in

this book unless your doctor tells you otherwise.

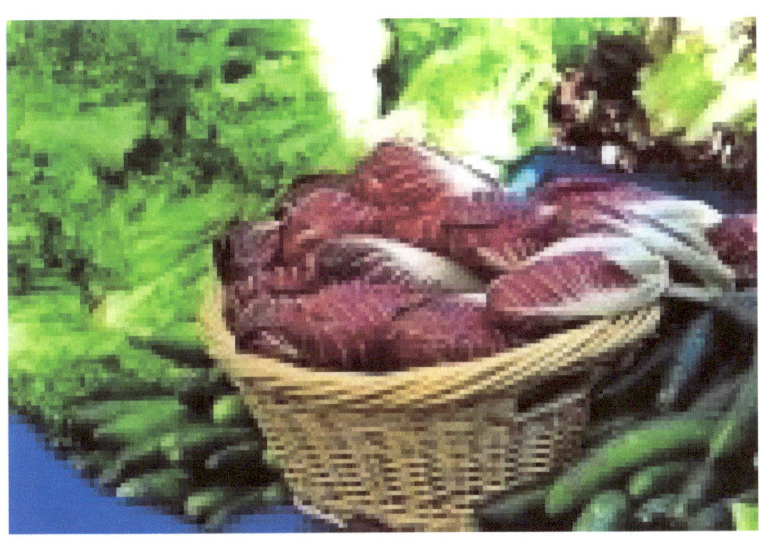

Prone to Arthritis?

Neutralize the pain within sixty seconds by

rubbing **"Castor Oil"** directly into the affected

area. Also, you can counter balance the effects of

Arthritis with some foods high in these nutrients:

CBD Oil

Coral Calcium

Vitamin E

Glucosamine and Chondroitin

Vitamin C

Vitamin A

Vitamin D

Juniper Berries

Boswellia

Medical Marijuana, Hemp Oil Extract or high levels

of CBD oil

Or get it here http://tinyurl.com/MedMariJane

Ginger

Turmeric

Black Strap Molasses

MSM Collagen

Alfalfa

Hyralonic Acid

Gelatin

You can also try this anti-inflammatory "Defense"

Here is the link:

http://www.lnk123.com/aff_c?offer_id=614&aff_id=193678 for those reading the paperback

version. Or try "Eazol" or "Joint Advance"

DAIRY

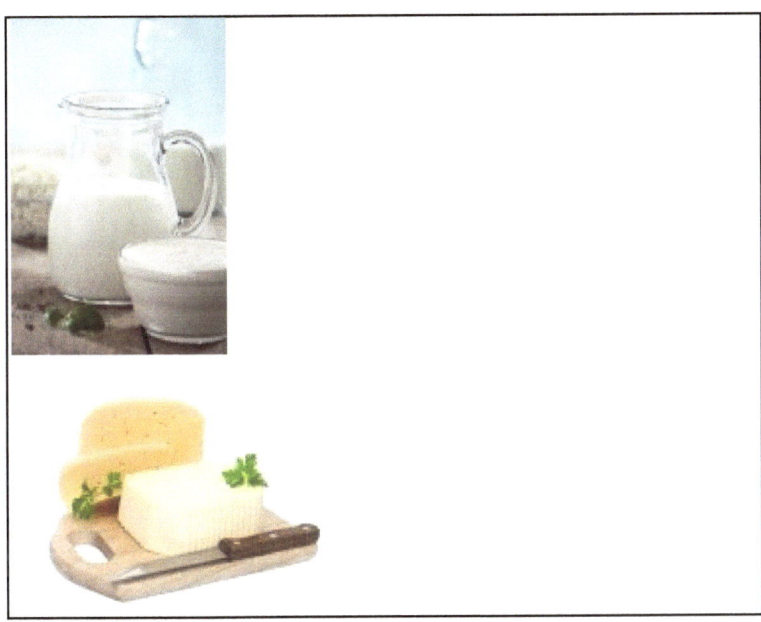

Dairy is a natural form of calcium. Although now they are saying that the phosphorus in the milk depletes the body of calcium and that we are better off getting our calcium from vegetables rich in calcium.

Try avoiding grains that cause inflammation. Inflammation is the cause of the pain in most cases. Bromelain Enzyme can be found naturally in Pineapples. Bromelain is an anti-inflammatory that really works fast on knee pain.

GINGER

Ginger is another great for an anti-inflammatory.

Try to keep your body at a Ph of around 6 for optimal pain relief. Be aware of which foods trigger your pain.

Chemotherapy Treatment Success Enhancers:

Ginger greatly decreases nausea in Chemo patients. Selenium before, during and after Chemo greatly increases the success rate of healing as well as greatly decreases the chances of the return of cancer.

 Gamma Vitamin E fights breast and prostate tumors.

Turmeric shrinks tumors

 IP6

Black Strap Molasses turns blood alkaline which greatly reduces the chances of cancer. Find most of the vitamins here "Health Buy Store".

 1 eight-ounce glass of water with ½ teaspoon of baking soda around 3PM each day.

1 eight-ounce glass of water with 1 teaspoon of

apple cider vinegar each morning upon awaking.

Garlic cleanses the cholesterol out of the blood

stream.

Dissolve Bone Spurs:

Acidic Calcium infused with K2

Find it here "Health Buy Store"

Chelation Therapy (Remove toxins build up):

Advanced Artery Solution

Saline Colonics

Colloidal Silver

Angio Prime

Omega 3

Lecithin

Garlic

COQ10

Vitamins D, E, & K,

Pomegranate Juice. (Compliments of Dr. Hans

Petermann)

Prostrate or Breast Cancer:

IP6

Gamma Vitamin E 400IU

Selenium

Turmeric

Black Strap Molasses

Schizandra

3 cups of Green tea per day decreases breast cancer by 50%.

2 aspirin per week reduces risk of breast cancer by 20%

Vitamin D decreases risk of breast cancer by 20%.

Anti-Inflammatory "Defense"

Recently it was reported that Pro football players are at greater risk of early Alzheimer's disease because of the multiple blows to their head. Obese African American women have greater risks and show symptoms of Alzheimer's much earlier than the other study groups. There are some wonderful natural ways to combat memory loss and stimulate brain health.

Brain Health:

Cumin and black pepper are good to detoxify brain tissue.

HGH

You can sprinkle turmeric on your eggs, along with sage, marjoram, basil, and garlic instead of salt.

Alzheimer's:

Ginkgo Biloba

Resveratrol

Pregnenolone

Vinpocetine

Coffee

Olive oil & Flax seed Oil

Cod Liver Oil

DHEA

Lecithin

L-Tyrosine

Rhodiola

Ashwagandha

Ginseng

Dl-Phenylalanine

Brain Health Continued on next page.......

Phosphatidylserine

Cumin

Black Pepper

[5HTP](#)

Lecithin is naturally found in eggs.

Erectile dysfunction or Impotence:

Ginseng

Deer Antler

Cayenne Pepper

L Arginine

Many drugs that are prescribed for depression will cause a loss of libido. Make sure that there is no strife between you and your spouse. Don't wander outside of your marriage and keep your priority on a good relationship.

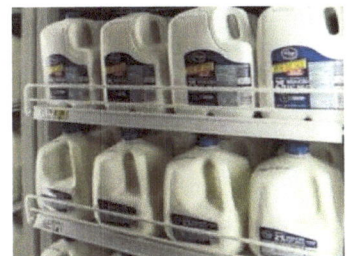

Bone Loss:

Coral Calcium

Collagen

Magnesium

Glucosamine and Chondroitin

Boswellia

Vitamin C

Vitamin D 3

Vitamin A

Vitamin E

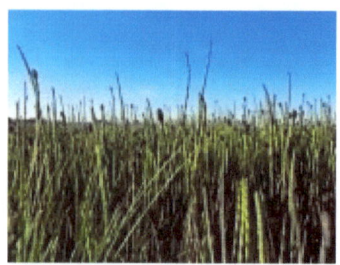

Cartilage Loss

Glucosamine and Chondroitin

 Collagen

Cats Claw

Horse Tail Herb

Vitamin E

Vitamin C

Calcium

Fibromyalgia:

Juniper Berries

Black Strap Molasses

Ginger is great for digestion and reduces

inflammation.

Turmeric shrinks tumors and fights inflammation.

Milk thistle detoxifies the liver.

Alfalfa turns blood level back to alkaline to reduce

arthritic pain)

Pineapple Bromelain to detoxify, digestive aid and an anti-inflammatory that works great on knee pain!

Tenninitis:

Cats Claw

Alfalfa

Black Strap Molasses (turns blood level back to

alkaline reduce arthritic pain)

Ginger

Pineapple or Bromelain (will detoxify and act as an

all-natural anti-inflammatory)

Chronic Fatigue:

B-Complex and Kelp

Plain Yogurt

Apple Cider Vinegar

Acidophiles (detoxify and anti-inflammatory)

Pro Biotics

Phosphatidylserine stops release of cortisol and helps with depression. Rest! A Stress free environment until complete health and wellbeing are restored for as long as necessary (depends on how chronic} It could take up to ten years in extreme cases where the immune system has shut down. Medical Science has proven that stress causes cancer. They have been teaching that in Modern Psychology since the early nineties. And they are still teaching it today in Social Science and Social Behavior Classes as I was a student of Psychology Holmes Community College Ridgeland, MS. In the early nineties and once again in 2011 I took another class on May 16, 2011 –

"Stressed to the Nines: The Hard Truth about Anxiety and You "

Constipation:

Cascara Sagrada

Senna

Wormwood parasite cleanser

Black Walnut Hull parasite cleanser

Slippery Elm

Old World Botanicals is a great place to find most everything mentioned in this book.

Esophagitis, Indigestion or Heart Burn:

Orange peel stops acid indigestion much faster and better than prescription ulcer medicine without the harmful side effects.

Licorice use like a sweetener in tea as a sugar substitute.

Bromelain

Aloe Vera gel

Apple Pectin or the skin of an apple.

Pain Management & Anti Inflammatory:

Medical Marijuana, Hemp Oil Extract or high levels

of CBD oil

Get it here: http://tinyurl.com/MedMariJane

Castor Oil (rubbed directly on the affected area)

Avoid Grains or any foods that trigger

inflammation

Ginger

Turmeric

Boswellia

Black Strap Molasses

Fish Oil or Omega Fats

Bromelain

Alfalfa

Anti-Inflammatory "Defense"

Yeast Detoxification:

Plain Yogurt on empty stomach

Apple Cider Vinegar

Pau D' Arco

Pro Biotics Oregano oil

Caprylic Acid

Beta Glucan

Here is another great place to get answers for

Curing Yeast http://kimig.tripod.com/yeastcures/

Parasite Cleansing:

Crushed Papaya seeds

Black Walnut Hull

Cilantro

Garlic

Worm wood

Earl Grey

Bergamot tea

Hair loss:

Collagen

Horse Tail

B-Complex

Vitamin E

Pine Bark

Exfoliate scalp with honey, sugar and conditioner; apply in circular motion let sit for fifteen minutes then wash as normal.

[Immune Deficiency](#):

Vitamin C

Selenium

Zinc

Colloidal Silver

Copper

Vitamin B Complex

Kelp

Vitamin E

Beta Glucan

DMG Mushrooms:

Maitake, Shiitake, Reishi,

Human Growth Hormone

Blue Berries

Grapeseed Extract

Manganese

Acai Berry

Dark Chocolate

Coffee

Co Q 10

<u>Hepatitis or other liver disease</u>:

Milk Thistle

Burdock Root

Hyssop Red Clover

Green Vegetables

Echinacea

Insomnia:

Collagen

Dong Qui

Valerian Root

Magnesium

Melatonin (naturally found in Milk, Turkey, or Chicken)

Melatonin

Stay away from caffeine after 12:pm noon, avoid herbs like Ginseng, Guarana, and Guta Kola after 11AM.

Wrinkle Reduction:

Natural Alpha Hydroxy ie apple juice, sugar, or honey & brown sugar applied to the wrinkles at bedtime.

Remove with Corn meal facial scrub in the morning. Use plain coconut oil to moisturize.

Dark Circle Removal :

1 drop of Sweet Orange combined with 5 drops of grape seed oil

2 Witch Hazel (also helps with swelling)

3 Shepherds Purse (dissolve in water then apply)

To reduce swelling around the eyes:

Use 1/2 teaspoon of Preparation H cream only (not the oily ointment) and be sure not to get it near or in the eye. Apply to effected area.

To help heal the blood vessels around the eye use

2 Arnica tablets dissolved in 1 tablespoon of water

apply one drop under effected eye.

Anxiety:

Lavender tea

Skullcap tea

Valerian Root

Magnesium

Dong Qui (take when needed or during

ministration)

Phosphatidylserine (stops the release of cortisol)

Himalayan lamp (but you must not have it by the

bed because the brain remains active around a

Himalayan lamp)

Blood Clots, Restless Leg Syndrome or Varicose Veins:

Horse Chestnut

Aspirin

Vinegar rub downs

Ginger

Garlic

Onions

Niacin

Fever Few

Schizandra

Shepherds purse

Butchers broom

Lumbrokinase (Chinese Earthworm enzyme that eats blood clots it is also great for allergies)

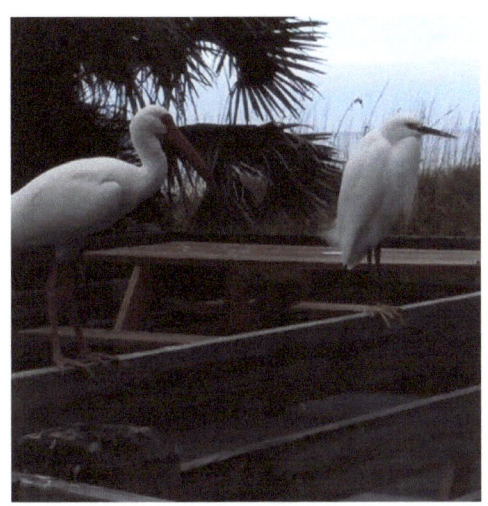

Poor Circulation:

Horse Chestnut

Schizandra

Aspirin

Hawthorne Berry

Fever Few

Niacin

Cardiovascular body movements.

Recently medical statistics revealed that people with poor circulation are at higher risk for heart disease and stroke. It is very serious and most heart tests do not reveal any problems in people with poor circulation when they are experiencing chest pain.

Be sure and see a medical doctor if you have chest pain. Butchers broom and Horse chestnut combined with Hawthorne Berry and Aspirin are more than enough to take the pain and inflammation away.

However, Hawthorne Berry is a very potent blood thinner and you must ask your doctor before taking it. You cannot take Hawthorn Berry prior

to having any surgical procedures.

Inflammation:

Ginger

Turmeric

Boswellia

Black Strap Molasses

Willow Bark or better known as Aspirin Bromelain

or better known as Pineapple

Anti-Inflammatory "Defense"

Fish Oil (Recent studies have linked inflammation

to heart disease and cancer)

(Click image to order anti-inflammatory

"Defense")

Sinusitis:

Xylitol nasal wash

Mullein

Olive leaf

Saline nasal wash (1 Quart of (distilled) water only, 2 tablespoons of canning salt 1 tablespoon of baking soda warmed to room temperature)

Bromelain

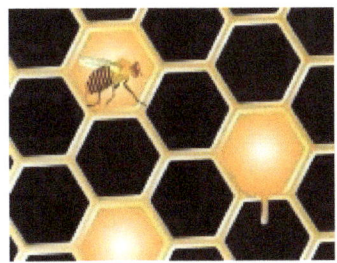

Allergies:

Bromelain

Mug wort

Bee Propolis

Mullein

Lumbrokinase (Chinese Earthworm enzyme that

eats blood clots)

Cholesterol Control:

Garlic

Ex. Virgin Olive oil

Niacin

Polycosanol

Remove all butter and vegetable oil from your food. Replace butter with Extra Virgin Olive oil for a spread on your toast or potatoes. And you can also use the olive oil in your salad dressings.

Switch to Coconut oil to cook all your food with.

This will eliminate bad cholesterol and help build up good cholesterol.

Heart Health:

CO Q10

Niacin

Garlic Fish Oil

Hawthorn Berry

Ribose

Horse Chestnut

Magnesium

Calcium

Ecotrin coated Aspirin

Polycosanol

Lumbrokinase (Chinese Earthworm enzyme that

eats arterial blood clots)

Recently medical statistics revealed that people

with poor circulation are at higher risk for heart

disease and stroke. It is very serious and most heart tests do not reveal any problems in people with poor circulation when they are experiencing chest pain.

Be sure and see a medical doctor if you have chest pain. Butchers broom and Horse chestnut combined with Hawthorne Berry and Aspirin are more than enough to get rid of pain.

Anti-Clotting:

Ginger

Garlic

Onions

Shepherds purse or soldier's tea.

Feverfew

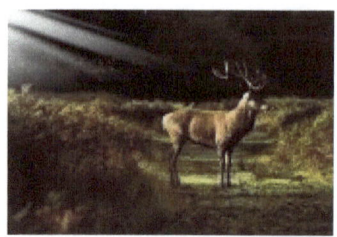

Deer velvet antler Has been scientifically proven

to provide the following benefits:

Combating Cancer

Improving the Immune System Functions

Improving Athletic Performance

Stamina and Strength

Improving Muscle Recovery from muscle stress

after exercise.

Also, an excellent natural supplement for

Women's Health.

Providing Vitality and Anti-aging properties for

Seniors.

Can be used as an alternative natural supplement

for Bodybuilding and Weight Training.

Has an excellent source of Growth Factors

including IGF-1 & IGF-2.

Improves and enhances sexual functioning for

both men and women.

It's a natural supplement for Arthritis.

Relieve Depression:

Phosphatidylserine

5 HTP

St. John's Wart

Turmeric

Dill

Marjoram

Saffron

Nutmeg

Peppermint

Everyone benefits in health and in weight control

when they switch ALL butters, vegetable oils, or

fat back grease and replace all of those with Olive

oil on toast, popcorn, salads, and switch to

coconut oil for cooking.

You must not cook olive oil at high temperatures

because it causes chemical structure to mutate

and instead of being healthy it becomes a health

hazard. On the other hand, Coconut oil can be

cooked at high temperatures and it is very healthy just as olive oils are.

You will also find that there are many sugar substitutes such as honey or Xylitol that is much better for your immune system and the Xylitol will help fight cavities while trimming your waist. It looks and feels exactly like sugar does.

Recently Medical Research has discovered that Chronic Inflammation greatly increased the risk for women in stroke and heart attacks or heart disease. There is a new simple test to determine how much inflammation is in your blood.

See your physician to see if that is something that you need now. There are simple anti-inflammatory herbs and remedies mentioned above.

You can also start your day out with pineapple for breakfast. The enzymes in the pineapple help to breakdown the protein cells in the walls of cancer formation.

These are just a few simple ways that we have seen to bring great improvement for health naturally after years of research.

We use homeopathic remedies, herbs, teas, and supplements. We believe that the best cure is from the Great physician and creator the Great God Jehovah.

And that He has given herbs and nutrients that help us to maintain health by obeying His word and taking care of our temples (bodies) by respecting them with good health care practices.

One thing we all need each day of our lives is health!

Many are over stressed in over drive and have taxed the immune system to the point that it is shutting down.

In some cases, their bodies have excreted so much adrenaline from the Adrenalin Gland till there is not anymore "fight or flight" Epinephrine

[Epinephrine - Epinephrine (also referred to as adrenaline;) is a hormone and neurotransmitter. It is a catecholamine, a sympathomimetic monoamine extracted from the amino acids: phenylalanine and tyrosine. (Referring to the adrenal gland, which sits atop the kidneys and secretes epinephrine) When this happens our body becomes vulnerable to disease.

This will keep causing the body to continual release cortisol. It will wear down the immune system. Cortisol is what causes women to have too much stored fat in the belly. And maybe related to the rise in heart disease in women. In some cases, it is nearly impossible to stop this downward spiral of destruction because the chemical has such a profound effect on our brains that in turn effects our entire lives. But even the worst-case scenario can find hope in providing the body what it must have to function properly.

Let us help you to regain control of your health! Using all natural and botanical herbs combined with common sense, daily supplements of vitamins, minerals, and a healthy diet are basics that get the body back on track to optimal health. Rest is essential for the healing properties to manifest speedily. And a healthy environment is also important to get optimal results. We use a Healing Approach to master Disease Control and operate in Preventive Health care as well as Traditional and

Conventional Medicine applied conservatively.

The Bible tells us that we are to obey our

physicians and we would never counsel against

your own doctors' advice. Most of our remedies

can be found the kitchen cabinets anywhere,

U.S.A.

And if there is a concern about a specific herb we

would ask that you consult with your physician.

Our goal is to help you feel better, look better,

and live longer! We only provide Natural and

Homeopathic Remedies. And for the most part,

our goal of optimal health is obtained best by

Preventive Health Care.

Natural Remedies are generally less expensive than prescription drugs, less side effects, and usually have more benefits than just healing a specific disease. For instance, the treatment for fighting cancer also fights inflammation.

These herbs in and of itself is not the cure. But combined with a healthy lifestyle pleasing to God and eating properly, that healing will be activated. There are some foods that must be abstained from and other foods that need to be partook of. It is like if you were eating foods with high calories and no vitamin or nutritional value, we need you to now do just the opposite, high vitamin, and nutritional value with very few calories. Spices and Teas are very beneficial in the healing process. In the Consultation, we can determine which ones

are best for you.